PRAISE FOR DYING FROM DIRTY TEETH

"Hundreds of thousands of our loved ones are living with, and sometimes dying from, painful and expensive conditions that could be ameliorated or avoided by adopting the sound win-win solutions proposed in this book by Angie Stone. *Dying From Dirty Teeth* is concise, accessible, and on the mark."

— JOHN J. DUBATS, DDS

"Angie conveys a compelling explanation of why poor oral hygiene is a long-term care facility's most expensive and life impacting problem. It is silent and usually unrecognized. Angie offers solutions. If this easy to read message got to every nursing home resident's family member and every decision-maker in Medicare and Medicaid, all nursing homes in the country would have a dental hygienist on staff. End-of-life care is financially crippling our country. The impact of the simple action steps she suggests could dramatically reduce the costs of hospitalizations related to diabetes, heart attacks, strokes, pneumonia, and others."

— CHARLES C. WHITNEY, MD, PRESIDENT AND FOUNDER OF 3RD ERA DENTISTRY

"A large segment of our continually growing elderly population is underserved, if not neglected, in an essential aspect of their health, their oral care. Angie, because of personal experience and devotion to the cause, confronts the   )k."

— JOEL J. WALDMAN, DN

"*Dying From Dirty Teeth* is   ights on shamefully neglected concerns. Angie Stone weaves personal narratives together with acknowledged facts and science. This potent combination is guaranteed to pack an emotional wallop. Most of us will recognize a personal connection. The title suggests and this book delivers. Dying From Dirty Teeth is far more than a roster of intractable problems. It is sometimes shocking, sometimes sad, but ultimately optimistic with a stirring call to action."

— JOHN PELDYAK, DMD, AUTHOR OF *SWEET SMART AND DENTAL HEALTH*

"People are absolutely dying too soon from dirty teeth and Angie Stone's book uncovers this ticking time bomb. Hear her warning and heed her call because this information will impact your aged loved ones right now and all of us sooner or later."

— CHRIS KAMMER DDS, FOUNDING FATHER OF THE AMERICAN ACADEMY FOR ORAL SYSTEMIC HEALTH

"Angie is passionate and to the point while explaining the strains and demands of the certified nursing assistant, and the abilities and restrictions of the dental hygienist. A tremendous amount of health care money could be saved, and time with our loved ones increased, with the collaboration of these two professions. It's time for people to stop looking the other way. It's time to stop trying to fix and repair oral and systemic issues that can be prevented. This book clearly explains how logical it is to embrace routine oral care services by dental hygienists as preventive health care."

— JENNIFER RINKER, CNA, RDH, BS

"Thank you, Angie Stone, for putting a spotlight on this abandoned population. We need to correct the void before anyone else becomes a victim of this absence of care."

— CAROL ROSZEL, RDH, BSDH

"Angie has written a wonderful book that can truly help open our eyes to how oral care can, and should, be delivered to our elderly loved ones when they are no longer able to do it for themselves. As a CNA myself I would love it if someone came in to help me deliver the oral care, allowing me to concentrate on other aspects of ADLs."

— **ANDREA MAVES, CNA**

"In Dying from Dirty Teeth Angie Stone has written about a subject that is an urgent wakeup call for us all. Angie helps us see in a clear and unambiguous manner how something so simple can have such a dramatic and deadly effect on our loved ones. She helps us see the problem and what to do about it. This book is a must read for anyone with elderly parents or have loved ones in our care."

— **TODD COHEN, PROFESSIONAL SPEAKER AND AUTHOR OF** *EVERYONE'S IN SALES*

"An audacious champion for our precious elders, Angie Stone reveals the formidable monster in the room. Her compelling message brings with it an empowering solution for families, caregivers and others seeking a difference."

— **ANNETTE WISE, RDH**

"Socks before oral health? As a clinician and human being, this book tugged at my heart strings. Thank you Angie for putting a face to the untold thousands who suffer each year and for helping us begin to understand how we might help. Your book helped me understand the jobs and criteria that often handcuff nursing home workers. "Access to care" should not be a buzz word. I know your work has begun to change lives and bring hygienists together who want to work with this "in need" population. Nurses and hygienists must come together and stop the dying from dirty teeth syndrome. Shame on the powers that be that create what seem to be unsurmountable roadblocks with no suggestion or thought into providing a working solution."

— LISA C. WADSWORTH, RDH, BS

"Angie Stone has taken her passion and is making it into an oral care movement to help our elders, particularly when they can't help themselves. I look forward to seeing this book on the best seller list and Angie on *The Ellen Show, The Doctors* and more. She will change the world with this book and her work."

— PATTI DiGANGI, RDH, BS

"Having been in nursing homes for various family members, I am excited to see this addressed by a professional who cares. Thank you and bless you Angie."

— PATTY DUBATS, DENTAL OFFICE MANAGER

DYING FROM DIRTY TEETH

Why the Lack of Proper Oral Care Is Killing Nursing Home Residents and How to Prevent It

ANGIE STONE, RDH, BS

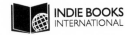
INDIE BOOKS
INTERNATIONAL

No part of this publication may be reproduced or distributed in any forms or any means, without the prior permission of the publisher. Requests for permission should be directed to permissions@indiebooksintl.com, or mailed to Permissions, Indie Books International, 2424 Vista Way, Suite 316, Oceanside, CA 92054.

Neither the publisher nor the author is engaged in rendering legal or other professional services through this book. If expert assistance is required, the services of an appropriate professionals should be sought. The publisher and the author shall have neither liability nor responsibility to any person or entity with respect to any loss or damage caused directly or indirectly by the information in this publication.

ISBN: 1-941870-11-2
ISBN 13: 978-1-941870-11-2
Library of Congress Control Number: 2015931105

Designed by Joni McPherson, mcphersongraphics.com

INDIE BOOKS INTERNATIONAL, LLC
2424 VISTA WAY, SUITE 316
OCEANSIDE, CA 92054

www.indiebooksintl.com

This book is dedicated to my mother-in-law, Gladys Stone, Grandmother Helen Schrantz, and longtime patient, friend, and supporter Ed Shaw. Without the needless suffering of Gladys and Helen and the opportunity to change that path for Ed, the vital message of this book would not have come to fruition. The three of them provide constant guidance from above. I feel their presence.

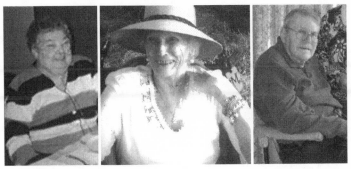

From left to right: Gladys (2003), Gram (2012), and Ed (2013).

TABLE OF CONTENTS

Foreword

The plight of the nursing home resident has been in the forefront of my mind for nearly two decades. As more people enter care facilities with more teeth, teeth with expensive dentistry, and an impaired ability to take care of their own oral health, palliative help for oral care must find a place in the facilities. As researchers find more system wide consequences from poor oral biofilm management and economists discover the true costs of poor oral hygiene, improvements in the status quo become even more imperative. Losing a tooth to poor oral hygiene, it turns out, is the least of the problem.

In this seminal book, Ms. Stone, lays it all on the line. Using cases she herself has experience with, she proves that things can be different. There are other hygienists in the land approximating what Stone is doing, but no one puts the same level of passion and the wherewithal to come out loud and strong offering solutions workable in today's word as well as offering solutions for the future.

Dental hygienists are highly skilled and motivated by clean teeth. They are women and men who signed up to work on the biofilm that accumulates on teeth. As a matter of fact, the profession of dental hygiene was invented to remove the debris on teeth so the dentists would have less work and could see the teeth he was about to work on. It seems odd that so many women have taken on the role of oral biofilm wranglers but they did. And most love their work. Ms. Stone shows us a workforce model that activates the vast number of dental hygienists who are currently under employed.

The message is clear, people with teeth live longer and people with teeth live better. There are many ways to die, some more dignified than others, but we all agree that dying from dirty teeth is not only undignified, it's wrong.

Thank you Angie Stone, RDH, BS for putting your facts and feelings into words on a page. Bring out your highlighter, oh gentile reader, you're going to need it.

Shirley Gutkowski, RDH, BSDH

February 2015

Acknowledgements

The thought of writing a book never even crossed my mind and now I hold my very own book in my hands. I certainly could not have accomplished this alone. Many people were instrumental in making this book a reality. Special thanks to:

Shirley Gutkowski for her ever present guidance and placing the idea in my head that I could write a book.

Beth Thompson and Shirley Gutkowski for having Michelle Prince as keynote speaker at CareerFusion.

Kris Potts for believing I had a book in me and dragged me almost kicking and screaming to Michelle's book writing conference.

Michelle Prince for an amazing Book Bound conference and book mind mapping experience.

Patti DiGangi for being a constant "connector" and introducing me to Henry DeVries and Mark LeBlanc.

Jennifer Rinker for spending her time and energy on being my personal proofreader and editor.

My long time employer, colleague, and friend, Dr. John Dubats, for seeing I was capable of more than providing dental hygiene services, for encouraging me to follow my path and being selfless in the process.

My husband, Jay, for his constant encouragement and support of my ideas and goals, even though he doesn't always know where they are going to lead. Also for dealing with the times I am in "Angie World."

My parents, Nicki and Jim, children Ashley and Spencer, brother Jim, and Aunt Andrea for always believing that I can do anything I decide to do and for always being there for me.

And of course, I would not be successful without the unconditional love I have received from each of these people and the countless others who have loved and supported me along my journey.

CHAPTER ONE

The Monster Problem

There is an epidemic going on among nursing home residents. This condition is making them sick and is leading to death. The situation has been happening for years; the problem is only getting larger, yet residents and family members remain unaware of it. Even the caretakers at nursing facilities are often times unaware of the magnitude of this issue.

Gladys became so physically ill with Chronic Obstructive Pulmonary Disease (COPD), at age sixty-three, she needed to move into a nursing home environment. As Gladys's oral health deteriorated, so did her lung health, or maybe it was vice versa, but the two conditions were definitely related. When the mouth is infected, the bacteria that cause the infection can easily be transferred into the lungs. This can compromise the health of the lungs and result in lung infections such as pneumonia. Couple this with lungs that do not work well due to COPD and the result can be deadly. Eventually Gladys's lung infections occurred closer and closer together. Each infection became harder and harder to resolve. The prescribed antibiotics got stronger and stronger. Eventually nothing more could be done, and Gladys lost her life to COPD. Or did she die from dirty teeth?

Ida broke her leg when she was 102 years old. It was logical to think this may be the beginning of the end of her life. Situations like this can often bring that on. But she recovered after three months of therapy. Shortly after that Ida contracted double pneumonia and she wasn't expected to make it, but she did. The antibiotics however had managed to kill off the good bacteria in her mouth and let the yeast take over. A yeast infection in the mouth is called thrush. Ida was in such pain she could not eat. She died of starvation. Or was it from the condition of her mouth?

Helen was placed in a nursing home. She was able to floss and brush her teeth, and was under the care of the nursing team and the nursing home dentist. She never had trouble with her teeth or gums. As her medications increased, her mouth became more and more dry. There are over 700 prescription drugs that cause dry mouth and she was on approximately seven of them. Even though she was legally blind and her body did not work well enough to allow her to walk, her biggest complaint was her dry mouth. The care team offered what they knew to address the problem, but it was not enough. When there is not enough saliva to control the bacteria in the mouth, teeth get cavities, and cavities need to be filled by a dentist. Helen was on Medicare. There are very few dentists who take this benefit for payment of services. As a result, the cavities were not filled. When teeth have cavities that are not filled, they break. As her teeth broke, her daughter would take her out to a private dentist for care, because a broken tooth was an emergency. Recommended treatment was always removal of the tooth in question. This was a vicious cycle, and one that no one, not the care team or the dentist, had any answers to. As a result, in the two short years Helen spent in the facility, she had lost 60 percent of the teeth she had managed to keep healthy for 90 years. She, like Gladys and Ida, had become a victim of our broken system of nursing home oral care and suffered needlessly from dental disease. Helen went to her final resting place with no front teeth, and cavities in the teeth that remained. While Helen did not die from dirty teeth, her dirty teeth certainly affected her quality of life. Can a poor quality of life decrease the will to live?

The Results from a Lack of Good Care

The lack of good oral hygiene is killing our elders and the ailment is completely preventable. Oropharyngeal bacteria are wreaking havoc. These bacteria can be controlled, and typically are controlled by most people through brushing and between the teeth cleaning. However, once people become dependent on others to remove these bacteria, the microbes run wild in the mouth, because they are not being kept at bay on a daily basis with tooth brushing and between the teeth cleaning.

The greatest risk of dying from dirty teeth comes when the bacteria in the mouth get aspirated into the lungs and the person contracts aspiration pneumonia. Aspiration pneumonia is a lung infection that is a result of oral bacteria, stomach contents, or both, being inhaled (aspirated) into the lungs. It is not unusual for small amounts of this material to trickle or be inhaled into the airway and into the lungs. In the general population the inhaled secretions have low bacterial count and are usually cleared out by normal defense mechanisms such as coughing. Bacteria are not allowed to reach the lungs to cause inflammation or infection.

This process is quite different with elders who have oral secretions containing high levels of bacteria and a compromised immune system. When an abnormally high amount of bacteria are aspirated and gain access to the airway, it can cause serious consequences. Elders cannot easily clear the microbes out of their respiratory tract. Bacterial pneumonias are strongly associated with aspiration of bacteria into the lower respiratory tract, which is normally a sterile environment. When this happens the result is aspiration pneumonia.

Infected and decayed teeth, as well as poor oral hygiene, have been correlated with the occurrence of aspiration pneumonia. Missing teeth and poorly fitted dentures predispose elders to aspiration by interfering with chewing and swallowing. When food is not properly chewed and swallowed it is allowed to remain in the mouth and break down. Aspiration of decomposing food that is laden with bacteria can lead to pneumonia as well.

Another issue our elders face in care facilities is oropharyngeal candidiasis or "oral thrush." This occurs when there is an over growth of yeast in the mouth. This also tends to be a minor problem in a healthy individual, but in the weakened immune system of a dependent adult, the symptoms of oral thrush may be more severe and difficult to control. Thrush occurs commonly in seriously ill and dying patients, but can occur in people of any age. Some of the risk factors for thrush include xerostomia (dry mouth), diabetes, use of antibiotics, dentures, and old age. A person who has thrush may not realize it until the outbreak is severe. At this point they notice pain, dysphagia (trouble swallowing), halitosis (bad breath), changes in the taste of food, diminished appetite, and reduced ability to consume food. The lack of taking in nutrition can lead to weight loss, eventual starvation, and death.

Even if elder care residents are not dying as a result of these masses of uncontrolled bacteria, they are suffering needlessly from cavities and periodontal (gum) disease because the bacteria in their mouths are being allowed to run amuck. When these bacteria cause periodontal disease, the destruction does not end in the mouth. A number of research studies show that teeth and gums burdened with the bacteria that cause periodontal disease can initiate cardiovascular disease, stroke, diabetes, and dementia. These bacteria can also complicate the control of existing diabetes.

Periodontal disease occurs when bacteria are allowed to thrive in the mouth and create a biofilm in which to live and do their dirty work. Once the body realizes the bacteria are doing damage, the immune system releases substances that inflame and damage the gums, the ligaments around the teeth, and eventually the bone that support the teeth. The body does this in an attempt to get rid of the bacteria. The release of these substances leads to swollen, bleeding gums, which are signs of gingivitis (the earliest stage of periodontal disease). If bacteria are not controlled at this point, the damage may continue resulting in full blown periodontitis (the advanced stage of periodontal disease) which is marked by loss of the bone around the teeth. This can cause teeth to become loose. Eventually teeth may be lost.

There are several causes of death that can be associated with poor oral health, including heart disease, stroke, diabetes, chronic obstructive pulmonary disease (COPD), and dementia.

Heart Disease: Several studies have shown that periodontal disease is associated with heart disease. Research has indicated that periodontal disease increases the risk of the development of heart disease. Scientists believe that inflammation caused by periodontal disease may be responsible for the association. The development of periodontal disease can also worsen existing heart conditions.

Stroke: Additional studies have pointed to a relationship between periodontal disease and stroke.

Diabetes: People with diabetes and periodontal disease may have more trouble controlling their blood sugar than diabetic patients with healthy gums. This appears to be a two way street. Those with periodontal disease are more likely to develop diabetes.

Chronic Obstructive Pulmonary Disease: Research has shown those with periodontal disease have a 60 percent higher likelihood of developing COPD than those without periodontal disease.

Dementia: Oral bacteria in the mouth due to poor dental hygiene have been linked to brain tissue deterioration.

Why Does Any of This Matter?

Elders, in general, have increased risk factors for heart disease, stroke, diabetes, COPD, aspiration pneumonia, and thrush. The lack of adequate oral care increases these risks significantly. While medical professionals go to great lengths to keep our dependent elders healthy, there is a huge piece of the puzzle that is not only in the wrong spot, it is completely missing. In the 2000 report, *Oral Health in America*, the U.S. Surgeon General pointed out that total health cannot be attained until oral health is improved. There needs to be a movement to end this epidemic. While death certificates do not list oropharyngeal bacteria as the cause of death, they are most certainly the origin of many illnesses that lead to death. There are many challenges and this problem can seem unmanageable, however the circumstances can be turned around so elders are not dying from dirty teeth. This needs to be done sooner than later. The population is aging and our baby boomers are going to be the next generation of dependent adults.

CHAPTER TWO

The Ticking Time Bomb

Consider these trends. Life expectancy in 1900 was a little over forty-seven years. Life expectancy in 2004 was just over seventy-eight years. Life expectancy in 2050 is projected to be almost eighty-three years.

In a short 150 years, the expected life span of humans will have increased by 43 percent. In fact, those over eighty-five are the fastest growing segment of the United States population and this group is projected to rise from 5.8 million in 2010 to 19 million in 2050.

At first glance, this may seem wonderful. Surely living a longer life must be better than living a shorter life. But living longer doesn't necessarily mean people are living well. In 2000, an estimated ten million people needed long term care services. That doesn't mean however they were receiving those services.

Here is the current landscape of the aging population and nursing homes, according to the most recent *National Nursing Home Survey* (2004):

- Five percent of Americans over age sixty-five live in a staffed facility.

- Fifty percent of people age ninety-five and older live in a staffed facility.

- Currently there are 16,000 nursing homes in the United States caring for over 1.5 million people.

Our baby boomer generation is aging. This is the generation of Americans born between 1946, just after the end of World War II, and 1964. They are the largest generation of Americans born in U.S. history. As a result of this generation, beginning in 2010, 10,000 people per day began turning age sixty-five and this will continue until the year 2030.

This translates to 3,650,000 people turning age sixty-five per year, which means there will be 73,000,000 people over age sixty-five in 2030.

If 5 percent of that seventy-three million people will be living in nursing homes that means 3.65 million people over age sixty-five will be living in nursing homes in 2030. This is over twice as many residents as there were in the survey from 2004. If this trend holds true, the United States will need twice as many nursing homes to care for our aged population in 2030.

Doubling the number of residents in care facilities will also double the number of people at risk for heart disease, stroke, diabetes, and aspiration pneumonia, especially if bacterial levels in the mouths of residents are not kept an acceptable level to ensure health. The amount of dental disease will increase as well, as the baby boomer generation has traditionally had better dental care and will enter facilities with more natural teeth than the preceding generations. Science, the dental community, and individuals have made great strides in the quest of ensuring teeth remain in place and functional for a lifetime. This should be a great thing, but for those people who end up requiring assistance with oral care, teeth can actually become a burden on their health if oral care is not performed effectively. Prevention of systemic disease in the nursing home population may be easier to achieve if residents did not have teeth. It has been thought by some that it might be a good idea to extract all teeth prior to admission to nursing facility. This of course is absurd and this solution does not come without issues. Removal of all the teeth adversely impacts nutrition and has a negative effect on self-esteem. If teeth are replaced with dentures, they also need to be cleaned effectively to prevent serious disease. Short sighted people could offer removal of teeth as an option if nothing is done to prevent the needless suffering from dental disease.

Dental Care of Generations (GI versus Silent versus Baby Boomer)

Current residents of nursing facilities tend to be from the "Greatest Generation," also known as the "G.I. Generation." They were born from around 1901 through 1924, and became adults during the Depression. This generation includes veterans who fought in World War II.

More and more folks from the next generation, "The Silent Generation," are becoming residents in nursing homes. This generation is also known as the "Lucky Few" and were born from 1925 until 1945. This generation also includes veterans of war, as the Korean War and the Vietnam War took place when these people were becoming adults. The children who grew up during this time worked very hard and kept quiet. They were raised in a time where it was commonly understood that children should be seen and not heard. As adults, this generation was good at taking direction, did not tend to rock the boat and often stayed at one job for forty-five years.

By nature of the economy, lack of knowledge about dental health, and lack of available dental technology while they were children, the GI Generation and the Silent Generation were not overly concerned with their dental health as adults. They just took things as they came. These generations typically went to the dentist when they had pain and the offending tooth was likely extracted. Extractions were customary because the procedure of endodontics (root canals) was not perfected, money was tight, and the world had not discovered how vitally important teeth are for quality of life. Spaces that teeth once occupied were left vacant, or were replaced with partial dentures. Once all teeth were lost, dentures were fitted. These generations grew up knowing they were likely to have dentures when they were old.

Technology to aid in prevention of dental decay was lacking for these generations. Any fillings that were placed were usually very large. Teeth can decay easiest around existing fillings, just as a car tends to rust again around areas that have rusted before, leaving this population prone to recurrent (reoccurring) tooth decay. Having not been taught the importance of cleaning between the teeth (flossing) and routine dental cleanings presents another challenge. These folks are at a higher risk for periodontal (gum) disease. All of these situations make the current cohort of nursing home residents' ideal candidates for acquiring dental disease. This is who and what caregivers are dealing with currently in the nursing homes.

The next group that will become nursing home residents is the Baby Boomer generation. This generation is widely linked with privilege. As a group, they had the most money, and were able to be more active and healthier than any generation before them. They were the first generation who grew up thinking the world they lived in would get better and better with time. The income they earned was greater than previous generations as well, which allowed them to have more things, such as designer clothes, bigger homes, and fancier cars. The Baby Boomers are often criticized as wanting and having too much. This generation also tended to think of themselves as a special generation.

The characteristics of the Baby Boomers are very different than the previous generations and so are their dental experiences. With an increase in income and insurance benefits came the ability to have regular dental check-ups and cleanings. Advances in dental technologies allowed the boomers to have dental disease treated earlier, which has resulted in the saving of teeth. When boomers lost teeth they were able to replace them with bridges that were permanently cemented onto remaining teeth on either side of the area where the tooth was lost. Full dentures in this group are rare and partial dentures are less prevalent in this group than in previous generations. Younger boomers are likely to have high-end cosmetic dental restorations in their mouths such as veneers, implants, and full mouth reconstruction.

The world needs to be warned: The next generations of nursing home residents are going to require more oral care to prevent the loss of teeth and irreversible damage to existing dental work. If oral care is not adequate, not only will dental health suffer, but there will be an increase in heart disease, stroke, dementia, COPD, and diabetes, due to having more teeth than ever before.

Dental treatment as Baby Boomers know it is usually non-existent in nursing facilities. Medicaid and Medicare pay very little, if anything, toward dental care and residents rarely have money left to pay out of pocket for these services. The days of having cleanings and dental checkups once someone is a resident in a nursing home are, in most cases, over. The best that can be hoped for is that the health of the mouth will be maintained. That too, becomes a challenge in the nursing home environment.

This is a recipe for disaster. More residents, more teeth, no money, no access to care, and no one to help preserve oral health has the potential to increase the numbers of people dying from dirty teeth. The country's dental and medical professionals are turning their heads the other way and refusing to see how a lack of oral health is killing those in one of the most vulnerable populations on the face of the planet—our beloved elders.

CHAPTER THREE

Sound the Alarm

It seems that oral health, something that appears so simple, should not be difficult to accomplish or manage. But for our elders, it is very difficult for many reasons.

A large issue for dependent elders is lack of access to traditional dental/dental hygiene services. The best scenario to keeping the population dentally healthy would be the ability to have care by dental professionals: routine check-ups and dental hygiene visits followed up by the treatment of any noted dental disease. However, there are several road blocks to this kind of care for this vulnerable group.

The sticking point with all problems tends to be money. Most dependent elders do not have cash or insurance benefits to pay for visits to the dental office. Medicare, which is federally funded, pays nothing toward dental services. Medicaid is a joint federal-state program, where federal dollars fund most of the program and each state has control of their own Medicaid dollars. This program typically pays very little toward dental care and benefits vary from state to state. There are some provisions for dental hygiene procedures for disabled folks who have Medicaid benefits, but most people do not know this. One legislator commented if all the people in nursing homes received the dental hygiene services they are eligible for under Medicaid, the Medicaid system would be bankrupt. No wonder no one knows services are available. This cannot be publicized if the system can't handle providing benefits that people are entitled to.

But there is another piece of the money puzzle. Even if a dependent elder does qualify for dental/dental hygiene services through Medicaid, it can be very difficult to find a dentist who will treat them and submit for reimbursement to Medicaid, as very few dentists in the United States are signed up to be Medicaid Dental Providers.

However, even if the majority of dentists were Medicaid providers, or if the elder had another way to pay for services, it can be impossible to get them to the office for service. Transportation is another road block. Dependent elders seldom have their own vehicles and if they do, it is likely they are unable to operate them. People who are not familiar with the nursing home environment may be thinking that the elder's family members could provide the transportation. That is a possibility only if there are family members available to transport during normal business hours. Private transportation is likely not possible. Many elders are unable to get into traditional private transportation. If they can get into an automobile, many autos are unable to transport wheelchairs, walkers, oxygen, etc.

Facility provided transportation can be an alternative to private transportation. While this seems like a good option, there can be barriers with this as well. Vehicles that can transport elders in wheel chairs are expensive and sometimes there is a charge to the elder for this service. If there is no money to pay, the elder cannot be transported. The elder may require a staff member to accompany them. It is not unusual for facilities to be understaffed, so they don't like to send people out with residents that are going off site. Also, to take residents out, especially if they are demented, is really very difficult and challenging. Getting them out of the facility, getting them into a vehicle, taking them to someone they don't know compounds their anxiety and dementia. Upon their return, the staff gets to deal with an agitated resident. The last thing care team members want is someone who will require more attention, especially if they are understaffed.

There may be some residents who have a way of paying and have transportation to get to the office. However, the challenges do not stop there. Dental offices and dental personnel are not always prepared to see elders with special needs. It is necessary that the office is handicapped assessable, which at this point in time, they should be. Offices that have been "grandfathered" in with the handicapped assessable laws are not accessible. If the resident arrives without someone to assist with transporting the resident to the dental chair, the dental team now is responsible for that transport. Dental professionals typically do not have any formal training with these types of transfers. If the elder needs to use the restroom and requires assistance, dental professionals are not trained in this process either. Risk of a fall in the dental office is great and if a medical emergency should arise there are no nurses available. A nurse would be most helpful in this situation due to their extensive training in initiating lifesaving treatment.

The bottom line is that for this population, traditional dental office visits are difficult, at best.

In-House Dental/Dental Hygiene Services

If elders can't get to the dental professionals, bringing the dental team to them is an option. There are many services that are provided on site in nursing facilities. There are some facilities that have dental services available, but it is not the norm by any means. When this service is offered there is typically a dentist and maybe a hygienist who visits the elders with mobile dental equipment. The equipment is usually set up in the beauty shop and treatment is provided there. This certainly reduces the expense and stress of having to get the elder out to the dental office.

The issue of money is still not addressed with this model. Many times the only residents who receive services are those who have signed up for dental services. This can come with an additional cost to the resident or their families. When being cared for under this kind of system, the services are not as comprehensive as one would receive in a traditional dental office.

While the resident may receive dental exams, dental needs are not tended to unless the resident is in pain. While providers of these kinds of services are well meaning, there are not enough of them to meet all the dental needs of this population. In addition, it is expensive to maintain all the materials and manpower necessary to take care of the extensive dental needs of nursing home residents.

Further concern comes with low compensation for the dental professionals who provide in facility dental services. This fact—added to the reality that this is a most difficult population to work with, quality dental equipment is lacking, and state of the art dental management systems nonexistent— deters dentists from wanting to serve this population. A career spent serving patients in a traditional office is more attractive for dentists. Who could blame them?

Despite the fact the masses of dentists opt to work in private or corporately owned dental offices there is a workforce who could serve this population and provide preventive services. This workforce requires less compensation than dentists, their services do not require as much equipment as dental services do, and there are a large number of these professionals who are not employed at all or are under employed. These professionals are the dental hygienists.

Nursing home residents who receive prevention based dental hygiene services are healthier but these services are rarely received by them because there are roadblocks in place that prevent these services from being delivered.

Access to Dental Hygiene Care

Dental hygiene services without any constraints, meaning that any registered dental hygienist (RDH) can have their own equipment and provide services in nursing homes, is not allowed in any state other than Colorado. There are many states that have laws in place to allow RDH's to enter into "collaborative agreements" or other arrangements with a dentist. States with these arrangements boast that they allow direct access to care from RDHs to elders in residential facilities. A close look at these laws reveals that every state with these provisions requires a dentist to be involved, at some point, in the treatment of the resident. These laws appear to be a great answer to dental hygiene access to care issues. In reality, however, these agreements often cannot be executed due to the lack of dentists who are willing to enter into these agreements. As a result, residents go without health preserving dental hygiene care. Out of 100 RDHs recently polled in Alaska, only one had entered into an agreement with a dentist. The regulations of having a dentist involved are roadblocks to dental hygiene services.

Dental hygienists are licensed professionals. They have gone to at least two years of school where they completed over 3,000 hours of didactic and clinical training. Candidates for the degree of dental hygiene are required to pass a national written board exam and a regional clinical exam to obtain a hygiene license. Requiring RDHs to have an agreement with a dentist in order to provide services to our vulnerable elderly population is simply a way for dental examining boards to control the interest of the dentists. Those interests are to ensure dentist involvement so they maintain control of the activities of the dental hygiene community. Other licensed professionals such as massage therapists, beauticians, nail technicians, etc., can provide services without others overseeing them. Dental hygienists should be afforded these same opportunities. They have earned it just as other professionals have.

As a result of these numerous challenges, residents are not being seen by dentists or dental hygienists. This means resident's oral health is in the hands of the care team: nurses and nursing assistants. But neither of these groups of professionals are the authority on the subject.

Chapter Four

Certified Nursing Assistant Oral Care Training

While Certified Nursing Assistants (CNA) are the ones providing oral care to dependent elders, the training they receive on this topic is next to nothing. Nurses have more oral health/oral care training than nursing assistants. However, even the extent of the education they receive on this topic is not sufficient to be able to provide adequate oral care, and nurses are not the ones responsible for actually providing this activity of daily living (ADL).

Nursing assistant textbooks are typically written by nurses and, due to their limited knowledge on oral health, this section of the text only focuses on brushing, flossing, and denture cleaning. Photos are placed in this section of how to do this correctly. The 2005 textbook, *Being a Nursing Assistant* by Francie Wolgin states, "Care of a person's mouth and teeth is called oral hygiene. A sick person's mouth often has a bad taste because of the medications or the illness. The tongue may be covered with a greyish coating that spoils the appetite. With good care the patient's mouth will feel fresh and clean and may increase the desire to eat." This discussion is all about eating because if residents lose weight in a nursing home, it is problematic.

Some textbooks recommend that teeth should be brushed every morning, every evening, and after eating, as well as flossed once a day to promote healthy gums. The idea that nursing assistants are able to brush every residents teeth three times a day and floss them once per day is absurd. If nursing assistants are able to get teeth brushed, it is not for a full two minutes, as recommended to remove all plaque/debris from the teeth. Facilities specifically train CNA to never put their fingers in a resident's mouth, therefore flossing rarely done. This expectation sets CNAs up for failure from the beginning. The first day on the job, when they are unable to accomplish everything, oral care gets omitted from the list. Oral care is easy to neglect because no one notices it hasn't been done.

In addition to a lack of information, nursing assistant textbooks are not providing up to date information on the topic. A popular textbook, *Lippincott's Textbook for Nursing Assistants* by Pamela Carter, contains the following information: "Keeping the mouth and teeth clean and healthy is an important part of personal hygiene. A clean, healthy mouth feels good and makes the food taste better, and contributes to overall health." This again reflects the importance of residents eating.

An early version of that textbook said, "Poor oral health can cause gingivitis which can lead to Pyorrhea." The word pyorrhea has not been printed in dental literature for decades. New nursing assistant graduates were entering the workforce having learned terminology that is completely outdated. For the record, the definition of pyorrhea is, "a discharge of pus, inflammatory condition of the peridontium. Also known as Riggs Disease." Today this condition is referred to as periodontal disease. Angie Stone and Shirley Gutkowski contacted the publisher and offered feedback on the oral care chapter. The latest version of the text now reflects the term periodontitis instead of pyorrhea.

Nursing assistants are also taught to tell the nurse if they see bleeding gums, broken teeth, or sores in the mouth. They are instructed to report any foul odor coming from the mouth. There are no photos in the texts of anything they're supposed to be looking for and many residents have issues with their teeth that nursing assistants would have no idea about. Expecting CNAs to report oral situations that they have never seen and have no education about is not a good practice. Remember that most of the time CNAs aren't even able to get in the mouth to look. Oral care is the task nursing home residents resist the most. This presents a challenge in and of itself. Nursing assistants do not have the training or time to properly deal with this behavior.

Oral care in CNA textbooks is put next to hair care. This location gives the impression that brushing and flossing teeth is cosmetic in nature. Lack of effective oral care can cause death. Placing education about oral care in the infection control section or wound care section would give oral care the attention it deserves and impress upon students its importance.

Approximately one hour of a 120 hour certified nursing assistant course is spent on oral care. In that hour, students are lectured to and expected to complete hands-on practice. Students practice on each other the same way as dental hygiene students do at the beginning of their formal education. CNA students are typically eighteen to twenty years old. Their oral health does not reflect the oral health conditions of residents, so they are not afforded the opportunity to see any conditions they have been asked to look for. They're cooperative with each other and if they simulate the resident behavior it's funny.

While practicing oral care on each other students approach their "residents" from the front. The toothbrush is held like a sword and the attempt to gain access to the mouth. With their fellow students, this approach works. It will not work with the majority of residents. When a resident turns their head because they don't want their teeth brushed the tooth brush is dislodged from the mouth and toothpaste is likely all over the resident's face. If the resident decides to spit, the CNA is right in the line of fire.

Students don't provide oral care on a real resident until their externship and there's nobody there teaching them how to do it. CNAs are on their own to do the best they can with the limited education they have received. Their first few experiences of providing oral care have the ability to form the CNAs opinion of oral care. Bad experiences will make them shy away from administering oral care for the rest of their careers.

Having a hygienist present up-to-date information in the classroom and offer tips during hands on practice is a realistic way to improve oral care education. Showing photos of what they can expect to see and teaching students to come from the side of the resident are two little things that can quickly improve the CNA experience of providing oral care. This process can make a CNA more comfortable with providing oral care and can directly impact the health of the people they serve.

Who Is The CNA?

Some people, especially dental hygienists, think nursing assistants do not do their jobs. This stems from the poor oral health situations they see in residents when they present for dental hygiene visits. It is wrong to assume CNAs are slacking because oral care is not adequate. CNAs are doing their job, but they cannot be expected to provide oral care to residents with the expertise of a dental hygienist. In addition to not having the training a dental hygienist has, nursing assistants have their hands full with a multitude of duties that need to be completed. Residents have situations that are a higher priority than getting their teeth brushed and flossed. Nursing assistants help with activities of daily living, i.e., eating, bathing, toileting, dressing, lifting, or helping the residents in or out of bed. Some are certified to administer medications. A successful shower can be something to celebrate, as nursing assistants wipe sweat off their foreheads. They provide emotional support to residents and for most residents they assume the role of their family. Many of the patients they care for, and get close to, pass away. The job of the CNA is daunting.

To make things more challenging, CNAs report it is not unusual to have twelve or more residents to care for at one time. Registered nurse responsibilities for each a resident take a half an hour per day on average. Licensed Practical Nurses (LPN) spend just over half an hour with each resident, while a CNA spends two hours with each resident. With this kind of workload, it is not shocking oral care does not get accomplished by nursing assistants.

When CNAs are asked, "If you have to accomplish oral care with a resident and put their socks on, but you only have enough time left to accomplish one of these things, which one will you complete?" They always answer the socks. When asked why they would choose this the answer is usually, "Because people will notice if the residents don't have their socks on." Absolutely nobody checks if the oral care is done. Nobody knows that's going undone and frankly no one seems to care. But a resident not having socks on their feet can lead to a reprimanded due to the high risk of falling.

There are formal education courses at technical colleges, but those who want to become nursing assistants are not required to go to school and work experience is not necessary. In some facilities, nursing assistants are not even required to have a high school diploma. On the job training is allowed. If the facility receives Medicaid and Medicare funding, nursing assistants are required to have seventy-five hours of training in the facility and pass a competency evaluation. In light of the rapid increase in the aged population there are going to be many more people requiring care. This translates into a 20 percent increase in CNA jobs annually.

Job turnover among nursing assistants is high and there are many reasons for this. The first issue is low pay. Salaries for CNA in the United States lie in the neighborhood of $11.54 per hour. Pay starts at $8.89 per hour and can approach $15.31 on the higher side. Limited advancement, poor management from employee relations, and difficulty of the work also contributes to high turnover rates. Facilities who deliver poor quality of care, where residents have more bed sores, and who use restraints, catheters, and mood altering drugs to keep the people manageable experience the highest turnover. More than 70 percent of CNAs change jobs in a given year. This is an excessively high turnover.

Given the items discussed in this chapter, the challenges CNAs face in their chosen profession become clear. They selected the profession because they wanted to help people. This is not different from the reason most people choose to become hygienists. Both groups dream of changing people's lives for the better and are on a mission to make the world a better place.

Nursing assistants need support in many areas and one of those areas is oral care. Hygienists have the ability to offer support in this area just as other professionals offer support in their area of expertise. For example, physical therapists (PTs) visit residents at least weekly to provide therapy. The CNAs are then expected, to the best of their ability and limited training; perform daily physical therapy with the residents. The PTs understand that the physical therapy the CNAs perform will not be as proficient as what they provide. The health care team acknowledges the importance of the profession/specialty of physical therapists in keeping the residents healthy and having a good quality of life. Likewise the PTs understand limitations of the CNAs' time and qualifications. Everyone works together for the good of the resident. This needs to be done with oral care in order to improve resident's quality of life through better oral health.

Chapter Five

Oral Care In-Service Training

In an attempt to improve oral health of residents, nursing homes have implemented mandatory in-service trainings on the topic. These oral care in-service trainings are required to be attended annually by nursing assistants. A disheartening fact is that research shows these lectures do not translate to improved oral health of residents. This may be due to the content of training sessions. However, more likely reasons are time constraints and limited hands-on training, which do not allow nursing assistants to accomplish the task of oral care well enough, or often enough, to improve oral health. Providing education, however, is never a lost effort. If a dental hygienist, an expert on oral care, delivers the training, there is a possibility of the hygienist becoming a resource for the facility regarding oral care. This in and of itself would be a positive outcome.

Oral Health In-service Training Topics

Oral care in service trainings are typically presented by a nurse in the facility. Oral care education received by nurses is focused around completion of brushing and flossing. It makes sense that this is what in-service trainings are centered on also. When a dental hygienist provides this training, they bring a new face to the team, new information about oral care, and excitement about the topic. This translates to better reception of the information and increased knowledge of the subject. There are many things a hygienist can teach that will help nursing assistants understand why they are so adamant about good oral health.

BRIDGING THE GAP: Dentistry is always talking about how the mouth is connected to the rest of the body and how medicine and dentistry need to work together to ensure healthier patients. Providing an in-service training is a great way to begin bridging that gap. A collaborative relationship between the RDH and the CNA is important. Having a hygienist provide the in-service training portrays a message about how hygienists can be a resource and support to the CNA.

MEDICAL ASPECT OF ORAL CARE: Dental professionals understand the links between oral health and systemic health. As we learned in chapter 4, education regarding this is almost nonexistent. Discussing associations between oral health and diabetes, heart attack, stroke, aspiration pneumonia, Alzheimer's, etc., is important. There is no need to go into great depths on this, but it is necessary to point the connections out. Improved oral care can specifically be tied to a reduction in aspiration pneumonia cases and diabetes that is more controlled, which directly reduces medical costs for these two conditions.

INFECTION AND INFLAMMATION: Describing that infection is infection, no matter where it is on or in the body, can speak volumes to nursing home teams. It is also important to explain that an area of infection doesn't just stay where we can see it. Infection can travel to other parts of the body. In the case of periodontal disease, this infection does travel to other parts of the body and leads to inflammation of other body parts. If we were able to lay the surface area of a mouth infected with periodontal disease end-to-end, the infection would be the size of the palm of an adult's hand. Periodontal infection doesn't mean anything to nursing assistants, but bedsores do. Facilities can be fined when patients have bedsores. Put a sore the size of the palm of a hand somewhere on a resident's body and it will get noticed and treated. A periodontal disease infection is as serious as a bedsore. However, it's more dangerous due to the fact it can't be seen and the medical team is not identifying it. Improving oral care can prevent systemic infection and inflammation.

DECREASING COSTS: Thousands of dollars per resident, per year, in down line medical costs can be saved if oral care is improved. Facilities are tight on money. In order for these much needed facilities to stay in business, they need to find ways to save money. Not only can costs be reduced to the facility by improved oral health, costs are also reduced to the resident by way of needing less dental care and fewer medical treatments and hospitalizations.

QUALITY OF LIFE (QOL): QoL can be improved by keeping people pain free. With good oral care the chances of a toothache decrease. Dependent elders are usually on some type of pain medication. Dental pain can go undetected until the pain is so strong it is no longer controlled by the medication. Once pain is detected, it is not unusual to find that the decay has spread into the nerve, and a root canal or extraction is necessary. Improved oral health can prevent diminished QoL by preventing tooth pain. Facilities want residents interacting with each other because it improves QoL. A clean mouth helps make people feel like socializing with others, while a mouth that has not been brushed can make people want to stay in their room and keep to themselves. Most people would not consider beginning their day around others without cleaning their mouth first.

MAL ODOR (HALITOSIS): Certain nursing homes have an odor. Oftentimes it's coming from the gases that are being given off by the mouth. Volatile sulfur compounds don't smell good. Simply providing better oral care can reduce the odor in nursing facilities.

Dry Mouth: More than 40 percent of Americans age sixty-five and older take five medications a day. More than likely, most of them cause dry mouth. Nursing assistants know the mouths of their residents are dry. What they don't know is why and what they can do to make their residents more comfortable. A dental hygienist can talk to the nursing team about the adverse oral side effects of chemotherapy and radiation. The hygienist can discuss products and ingredients, such as xylitol, that help keep the mouth moist, therefore, improving oral health.

ROOT DECAY: Dental professionals know people don't get "long in the tooth." They know that the tissues recede and the roots are exposed. Many nursing assistants don't realize this. Hygienists also know that roots decay faster than enamel. Improving oral care plays a significant role in reducing root decay.

GINGIVITIS AND PERIODONTAL DISEASE: There is no need to provide an in depth discussion about the differences about these two diseases, but a basic discussion helps the nursing assistants understand what they are trying to prevent in the mouth. Simply explaining that gingivitis is the inflammation of the gums and periodontal disease is the loss of the bone, offers information they likely not have heard before.

PARTIAL AND FULL DENTURES: It is important to teach the nursing team that the resident's name should be on these prosthetics. Dentures and partials need to be kept clean. Food that is allowed to sit under these devices begins to decompose. This food gets aspirated into the lungs causing the resident to acquire aspiration pneumonia. This process can be deadly for a dependent elder.

Easy Ways To Address Oral Care

The following information is truly what nursing assistants are interested in learning about. These topics need to be included in an in-service training.

Individualized Daily Oral Care Plan: Oral care should be individualized just like many other aspects of a residents care. If a resident would rather have their teeth brushed at noon instead of eight o'clock in the morning this should be listed on the individualized oral care plan. Other items that should be listed are if the resident is cooperative with oral care, what special oral care products should be used to assist with this care, and anything that the resident does not like when providing oral care.

It is best when the nursing assistant and dental hygienist can discuss this care plan together. The aide will usually know what the resident is and is not capable of, while the hygienist knows what to recommend based upon the needs of the resident.

POSITIONING: Instruct the nursing assistants to approach the resident from the side, not from the front. Once the resident is in this position, the nursing assistant should place their arm over the resident's head and place their hand around the resident's chin. This provides head support for the resident and enables the nursing assistant to control any rapid head movements. When the nursing assistant is in this position they are not going to get spit on.

TOOTHETTES: These sponges on a stick are better than nothing. They are typically used to moisturize the mouth. They can be used as a toothbrush if there is no brush available. If using it as a toothbrush, the toothette should be used vigorously on teeth. Keep in mind, if used in this fashion, the handle is likely to bend. Using toothettes that are uncoated are better, as the usual coatings can cause mouth dryness.

BRUSHING: Brushing teeth can be a challenge for nursing assistants because many residents clench their teeth together and purse their lips. Teaching nursing assistants that this a good thing can change their whole attitude about oral care. Sliding the toothbrush in between the lips can be accomplished fairly easily while allowing the resident to clench. Cleaning only the fronts of the teeth is better than nothing, and is almost as good as brushing the whole tooth! Most biofilm accumulates on the facial (lip side) and buccal (cheek side) surfaces, while very little biofilm attaches to the lingual (tongue side) and occlusal (chewing) surfaces. Removing the biofilm on the facial and buccal surfaces can decrease the biofilm by more than 50 percent. Reduction of this amount is far better than not attempting any brushing because the resident is clenching. Oral care is not about being perfect, it's about getting the toothbrush in there and moving it around however possible.

If the growth of the plaque is disrupted every twenty-four hours the resident's oral health will improve. This is why it's vital for brushing to be scheduled once per day. It is more important to instruct the aides to get the brush into the mouth and do the best possible, rather than teaching them about the proper 45 degree angle. Remember, they are not dental hygienists, and cannot be held to the standard that a hygienist is held to. Teaching this to nursing assistants relieves some of their stress and allows them to focus on the best biofilm removal they are able to achieve on a resident once per day.

TOOTHPASTE: Apply a small amount of toothpaste on the brush. Generally a pea size amount is adequate. There is no need for the large amount of toothpaste that people usually use; this is unnecessary, causes excessive foaming, and generates the need to spit. When this happens with residents, they may spit at any time, causing the nursing assistant to be contaminated by this bodily fluid. Reducing the amount of toothpaste used eliminates the need for spitting and even rinsing. Toothpaste can be left in the mouth and swallowed, when small amounts are used. When fluoride is left in the mouth, and not rinsed out, it has oral health benefits. The biggest reason toothpaste is recommended is due to the fluoride it contains. It is okay not to use toothpaste if it becomes too difficult to manage the foaming, rinsing, and spitting.

XYLITOL: The magic of xylitol with any vulnerable population will improve their oral health by leaps and bounds and it is easy to get people to use xylitol products. When xylitol is consumed by disease causing oral bacteria, these bacteria cannot digest it, which leads to a reduction in acid production and eventual death of the bacteria. This process creates an environment in which non-disease causing bacteria can create oral health. Xylitol also stimulates salivary flow, which helps those with dry mouth. More saliva means more enamel healing. Chapter 6 provides a more in depth discussion regarding xylitol.

CHAPTER SIX

Xylitol and Professional Weekly Oral Care

With all the challenges CNAs face on a daily basis, oral care is often forgotten or avoided. Not only are CNAs strapped for time, oral care is a difficult task for them. Some of the reasons for this were discussed in Chapter 4, but there are other reasons for this as well.

Residents can be resistant to oral care. It is not unusual for residents to clench their teeth, move their head, spit at, or attempt to bite the caregiver. Once a nursing assistant has experienced being bitten, they tend to shy away from brushing and flossing residents' teeth. As a result of these time-consuming resistant behaviors, oral care is not attempted on a regular basis. While the average person would never consider going days without brushing their teeth, this can be the reality for nursing home residents. Fortunately there are ways to improve the elders' oral health that, when performed, will take the pressure off nursing assistants. These alternative methods will also improve elders' quality of life by allowing the proper professional to care for their needs.

Xylitol

The natural occurring sugar substitute, xylitol, has been proven to reduce the incidence of tooth decay and improve oral health. Xylitol is available in a variety of products including, but not limited to, gum, mints, candies, mouthwash, toothpaste, oral mist, mouth spray, and oral gel. With all these options available it is easy to get into the mouths of just about anyone. The train of thought is after each meal we encourage people to put xylitol into their mouths.

Xylitol was discovered in 1891 by the German chemist, Emil Fisher. He discovered it by accident while working with plants in his lab. As it turns out, it was a great discovery for health. During World War II there was a sugar shortage in Finland. They began sweetening their foods with xylitol since they couldn't get sugar. After the war, sugar became available again and wide spread use of xylitol stopped. An interesting thing happened when the epidemiologists began to look at tooth decay rates some years later. The decay rates in Finland were lower than decay rates in any other country. Everyone was perplexed by this, but they ultimately were able to figure out that the decay rates were lower in Finland because of the country's use of xylitol.

Widespread use of xylitol became practical in 1970, with the first chewing gum being launched in Finland and the United States in 1975. Since then there have been a few thousand clinical and laboratory studies that have demonstrated xylitol's preventive and therapeutic benefits. An interesting thing to note is that xylitol has many other uses, in addition to improving dental health.

Regarding dental health, xylitol is beneficial because it wreaks havoc on *streptococcus mutans* (*S. Mutans*). In dentistry we understand it is the *S. Mutans* bacteria that are the main culprits in creating dental disease, especially tooth decay. When *S. Mutans* ingest the simple carbohydrates (sugars) we consume they use them as a food source. The bacteria digest the sugar, which is always followed by secretions being released from the bacteria. These secretions are acidic and sticky. As we eat more sugar, this process is repeated and, before we know it, a biofilm has been formed on our teeth and gums. People often refer to biofilm as plaque. This can lead to a breakdown of enamel which leads to tooth decay and inflammation of the gums which can lead to periodontal disease. The traditional way to keep this biofilm off the teeth and gums is through brushing and flossing. The dependent elder population, however, is often times not able to remove this biofilm through this process. The dental profession has always thought mechanical disruption of the biofilm was the only way to control the biofilm. Thank goodness for our dependent elders, brushing and flossing is not the only solution.

When S. *Mutans* consume xylitol, the whole chain of events just discussed is disrupted. Xylitol cannot be digested by S. *Mutans*. Without digestion, there are no secretions, which in turn means there is no acid produced. So, essentially there is no development of an infectious, sticky biofilm. The inability of the S. *Mutans* to digest xylitol also leads to eventual death of these bacteria. Over time, the use of xylitol decreases the population of S. *Mutans* bacteria that reside in the mouth. This creates an oral environment in which bacteria that encourage dental health are allowed to thrive.

In addition to stopping acid production from the S. *Mutans*, xylitol increases the flow of saliva. Many elders experience dry mouth, which can lead to tooth decay. Improved salivary flow helps elders feel more comfortable, be able to eat easier, and sleep through the night. More saliva translates to an increase of calcium and phosphates in the mouth. These minerals assist with remineralization (enamel healing) of demineralized (broken down) enamel. This helps prevent tooth decay.

The use of xylitol after eating decreases sugar clearance time, the time sugar remains in the mouth to be consumed by bacteria. When the consumption of food stops, the pH of the mouth is acidic. Research shows it takes the body twenty to thirty minutes to bring that pH back up to neutral. When xylitol is put into the mouth after eating, the pH is back to neutral within five minutes. Reducing the time the mouth is acidic from thirty minutes to just five minutes, translates to a decrease in demineralization time by 75 percent. All of this can be accomplished by simply putting xylitol into the mouth for five minutes after eating.

This can be achieved by simply chewing gum, sucking on mints, applying tooth gel to the upper front teeth, or a series of other simple applications. There is no need to mechanically touch all areas of the teeth and gums to remove the biofilm. It is truly magical for those people who are unable to brush and floss effectively. Especially those who don't have people who can accomplish this activity of daily living (ADL) for them.

Professional Weekly Oral Care

Dental hygienists are the authority on oral care. It would be next to impossible to have a dental hygienist providing oral care on a daily basis for residents. However, it is possible to have a dental hygienist provide oral care weekly for residents. Research states professional weekly oral care can be an important strategy in reducing the incidence of aspiration pneumonia. Another research project states that professional weekly oral care can reduce the number of days residents have a fever and can improve oral health.

This procedure is through brushing and between the teeth removal of plaque with over the counter items, once a week. A dental hygienist performs this ADL. A hygienist is more than familiar with placing items into a person's mouth, so getting a toothbrush into a mouth is typically an easy task for a hygienist. Hygienists also know what they are trying to remove, are able to notice things that may not look right, and can report any findings to nursing staff and/or family members. Oral care is the only task they are providing, so they have time to spend accomplishing this task. A hygienist is the perfect oral care specialist (OCS). No specialized training is necessary, and no work force needs to be created. The facility and residents benefit by having experienced hands and eyes providing the oral care needs of the residents.

Chapter Seven

Case Studies

The dental benefits of xylitol are well documented in the literature. Most of the research has been done with children. It makes sense, however, if xylitol can reduce dental decay in children and improve their oral health, that it could do the same in dependent elders. Shirley Gutkowski, RDH, BS, FACE and Angie Stone, RDH, BS wanted to put this theory to the test, so the two designed, implemented, and completed the following twelve week study.

Case Study 1

This study was conducted in a nursing facility in Janesville, Wisconsin from November 1, 2007 through January 31, 2008. The study and the results were published in the November 2013 edition of *Integrative Medicine Clinicians Journal*, which is a peer reviewed medical journal. The full paper can be found on the IMCJ website.

There were twelve residents involved in this study. Six of them received the intervention of xylitol, while the other six received no interventions. The residents who participated were able to use the xylitol as directed by the nursing assistants.

The study was kicked off with an in-service training with nursing assistants in attendance and continued for twelve weeks. The CNAs were asked to have residents chew two pieces of Spry 100 percent xylitol sweetened gum or suck on three Spry 100 percent xylitol sweetened mints, depending on their individual care plan. The gum or mints were administered twice a day by the CNA. Once while they were dressing the resident for the day, and again while they were getting the resident ready for bed.

The CNAs were also asked to apply a pea size amount of MI Paste to the resident's finger and have them smear the paste on their teeth after lunch and dinner. MI paste contains Recaldent, a special milk-derived protein that releases calcium and phosphate to the surface of the teeth. The paste was added to the regimen in an attempt to create acid resistant enamel, and to give palliative relief for dry mouth.

Totals	AM: Xylitol	Lunch: MI Paste	PM: Xylitol	Bedtime: MI Paste	Total Missed Interventions	% of Interventions Missed/Person
Resident 1	2	11	12	14	57	10%
Resident 2	4	20	20	18	85	16%
Resident 3	4	20	39	40	126	23%
Resident 4	9	19	45	41	154	28%
Resident 5	15	35	23	20	125	23%
Resident 6	19	17	23	36	127	23%
Total missed	53	122	162	169	676	
% missed	10%	22%	30%	31%		

As can be seen in the chart, the compliance rate was over 70 percent for the three month study period. That is an impressive outcome. Research that has looked at teaching CNAs about brushing and flossing residents' teeth has never reported a 70 percent compliance rate. The nursing assistants were not taught anything about tooth brushing or flossing. They were simply asked to continue to do whatever they were currently doing for oral care.

Each resident had their mouth disclosed with two-tone disclosing solution. Biofilm that has been on the teeth for longer than twenty-four hours stains blue, while new biofilm (plaque that's been on the teeth for less than twenty-four hours) stains red. Photos were taken at the beginning of the study, at the six week mark and at the end of the study. Study photos can be viewed at www.hylifellc.com/studyphotos.

Resident one is schizophrenic. He never allowed anyone to brush his teeth. That is why there was so much blue staining in the initial study photo. The reduction in the biofilm is amazing over the twelve week period, and this resident was the least compliant of all the residents.

Resident two is a Vietnam War veteran. The CNAs did not want to take care of him because he smelled so bad. This was not discovered until the six week photos were being taken. The nursing assistants came to the researchers said, "We cannot believe how much better he smells." Prior to the use of the xylitol CNAs would cringe at the thought of having to be around him due to his odor. Now they could tend to him without smelling a bad odor from his mouth.

Resident three had basically no biofilm left in the last photo, except along the gum tissues of two teeth. However, even the tissues in these areas are looking better. Had the study continued for another twelve weeks, that biofilm would likely be gone.

Resident four had a great reduction in biofilm. Watch as the flora goes from blue, in the first photo, to red in the third photo.

Resident five's photos also show the biofilm changing color. It is obvious that no one was using any floss on this resident by the amount of biofilm still between the teeth.

This project certainly showed that xylitol can reduce the bacterial load in the mouth. This research was not intended to be an end all, be all, of anything. It was intended to show results with the hope that someone, who is more research savvy and has more resources, would continue to study the effects of xylitol on dependent elders' oral health.

Case Study 2

After seeing the research stating professional weekly oral care can improve oral health and create healthier dependent elders, Gutkowski and Stone designed and completed a second study, combining xylitol and weekly care. The project took place in four facilities in three states and included forty-five dependent elders. Each resident was given two Spry 100 percent xylitol sweetened mints after each meal, and they received brushing and flossing services once per week from a dental hygienist.

Each resident was disclosed with two tone disclosing solution, as in the first study, in the beginning of the study, at the six week mark, and at the twelve week mark. Each resident was placed in a category based on the amount of biofilm on the teeth. The categories were minimal, mild, moderate, and severe. Study photos can be seen at www.hylifellc.com/studyphotos.

The minimal biofilm category is defined as: No or very little red staining in initial photo. Oral hygiene is classified as good. No subjects began in this category.

The mild biofilm category is defined as: Several to most areas stained initially red, no or few areas of blue staining. Oral hygiene is classified as fair. Five residents (11 percent) began in this category.

The moderate biofilm category is defined as: Mixed areas of red and blue staining in initial photo. Oral hygiene is classified as poor in initial photo. Thirteen of the forty-five subjects began in this category (28.9 percent).

The severe biofilm category is defined as: Most stained areas are blue. There are no or very few areas of red staining. Oral hygiene is considered terrible and/or there are obvious visual signs of gingival inflammation. Twenty-seven of forty-five subjects began in this category (60 percent).

During the twelve weeks, 31 percent of the residents moved into a category of less biofilm.

BEGINNING

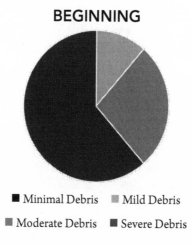

■ Minimal Debris ▨ Mild Debris
▨ Moderate Debris ■ Severe Debris

COMPLETION

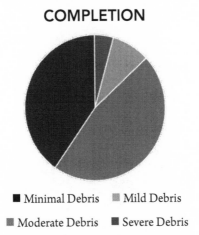

■ Minimal Debris   ▓ Mild Debris
▓ Moderate Debris   ■ Severe Debris

While not everybody had enough of a biofilm change to be categorized a category of less biofilm, 78 percent of the residents showed visual improvements of less biofilm.

CHAPTER EIGHT

Benefits to the Dental Community

Residents, family members, caregivers, the medical community, Medicaid, and insurance companies are among the groups that can benefit from improved oral care of our dependent adult population. There is one remaining group that has not been discussed, and that is the dental community.

At first glance, it is easy for dental professionals to dispute the concepts presented. Minds shift toward loss of revenue for the dental office, loss of supervision of dental hygienists, and proper adherence to practice acts. These items seem to always be at the forefront of thoughts in dentistry. If, however, the model offered is contemplated with open minds, it becomes apparent these concerns are not founded, and certainly do not take into consideration the health and welfare of the vulnerable dependent adult population.

Dental professionals are a vital component of the health care team. Patients who receive routine dental care can have that care delivered in the same dental office for ten, twenty, thirty years or longer, depending what point in the dentist's career patients join the practice. Patients grow older with the office. They entrust the care of their children and possibly grandchildren to the clinicians who have served them well. Patients are loyal to the dental team, and the dental team is loyal to them.

It can be worrisome for dental professionals to care for the aging patients they have become close to. As these patients get older their physical changes dictate variations in care. Clinicians do the best they can to manage these challenges. Elders are not able to sit for the length of time required to complete ideal restorative work and hygiene treatment. As a result clinicians can find themselves attempting to shorten treatment time to keep patients comfortable. Aging patients also are not always able to lie in a position that allows proper access to their mouth. The dental team provides care while standing, leaning, or hunching, which can be detrimental to the health of the professional. This is where the weekly prevention an OCS can provide is key to the elders' health.

Once a patient is unable to physically get to the dental office, the care team loses touch with them. This is when oral and systemic health begin a downward spiral. Dental offices are at a loss as to what to do to stop this from happening when they have no ability to provide services. The best they can hope for is that there is a dental professional tending to their patients' needs where they live, which is usually not the case.

Having a dental hygienist tending to the oral care needs of these precious patients provides a lifeline between the patient and dental office. The hygienist can relate any potential issues they see to family members or care teams, just as the nursing assistant is asked to do. The only difference is a hygienist knows firsthand what they are looking at. Family members know who the dentist of record is and can be asked to contact the dental office to see what the dentist recommends if there are any issues. The hygienist not only brings a skilled set of eyes, they can also communicate what they see to the dentist in terms that help the dentist understand what is going on. If the dentist wants to see the situation, the hygienist can send a photo of the item in question to the dentist.

If the dentist opts to see the resident, the hygienist can assist the family or facility in coordination of transportation. All of these tasks are things care teams do not have time to do and family members may not have time or know how to do. Hygienists can also ask family members if there happens to be any dental insurance or another way available to pay for dental treatment. Communication with dental offices has the ability to keep the dental team connected with long time patients.

This can also bring revenue into the offices, if residents have the ability to get to the office and pay for services. While these kinds of residents are not the norm, those who can receive and pay for services deserve to have that option.

In 2006 there were 286 accredited dental hygiene programs. The American Dental Hygienists Association reported 332 programs in 2013 and more programs continue to be developed. Compare this with the American Dental Associations statistics of just forty dental schools in the US and it is easy to see the numbers of hygienists far outweigh the number of dentists. Most dental hygiene programs are two years in length. A dental degree requires four years of undergraduate courses and four years of dental school. This difference in time of education also leads to over saturation of dental hygienists. As a result, many hygienists are underemployed or unemployed.

The existing workforce of hygienists can make a dramatic difference in the health of nursing home residents. Providing oral care for these individuals can provide meaningful jobs for those hygienists who are not adequately employed and afford them the opportunity to utilize their existing skill set. This, of course, is a benefit to hygienists. It can be a benefit for dental offices as well by reducing the number of hygienists who are practicing clinical dental hygiene but would like to be doing something else. This would provide positions to those who truly want to be working in the clinical environment.

Some dental professionals believe when dental hygienists provide oral care services, brushing and removing plaque from between the teeth, they are practicing dental hygiene. This belief brings up questions regarding the legality of this service. The concern is that in order to carry out this task, the dental hygienist has to follow the governing states dental practice act, which as discussed earlier requires involvement of a dentist in all but one state. Attorneys that have been consulted on this topic don't see a concern. The act of brushing and flossing teeth is not the practice of dental hygiene. People all over the world do this on a daily basis and even complete this task for others. Mothers and fathers, daughters and sons, grandmas and grandpas are just a few people who assist with oral care. Personal care workers are hired to assist with ADLs, which include the brushing and flossing of teeth. Nursing assistants are tasked with completion of this ADL with next to no education on the topic. Where does this thought that the rendering of brushing and flossing is the practice of dental hygiene come from?

Some state dental associations have told organizations that hygienists can deliver the services of brushing and flossing, denture cleaning and education, but they are not allowed to bill for these services. This is proof that it is not the service of helping this vulnerable population maintain optimal quality of life that is in question, but rather a question of someone making money other than the dentist. Recently the Federal

Trade Commission (FTC) has counseled organizations regarding such laws stating they are a restraint of trade. Some of these cases were presented by the FTC at the 2014 annual session of the American Dental Hygienists Association. These restrictions will not be allowed forever. Times are changing.

Until these restraints are lifted and there is no question if a hygienist can legally brush and floss the teeth of the elders and receive compensation, dental hygienists associated with HyLife, LLC, will maintain a caregiver certification. Caregivers are allowed to provide the ADLs and get reimbursed for their services. A professional who is both a hygienist and a care giver, who provides oral care is a benefit to everyone involved with the care of elders: those paying for care of the elders, medical professionals trying to control systemic disease of the elders, dental professionals concerned with the health of the elders, and most importantly, the elders themselves.

CHAPTER NINE

Funding Oral Care

In the first quarter of 2014, health care spending rose 9.9 percent in the first quarter, according to the U.S. Commerce Department's Bureau of Economic Analysis. This was the largest quarterly increase in more than thirty years. With such a large increase in spending, Medicare, insurance companies, nursing homes, elders, and their families are trying to find ways to cut costs. At first glance it would seem counterproductive to make funds available for oral care. A more in-depth look reveals just the opposite.

Medicare

In 2009, $484 billion was spent on mandatory Medicare payments. That number is projected to be $885 billion by 2018, according to the Congressional Budget Office. The

Medicare crisis is a topic often discussed by elected officials and citizens alike. There is talk that at some point Medicare will be defunct. In order to ensure Medicare's longevity money needs to be saved. Improved oral care, resulting in improved oral health is a way to save precious Medicare dollars.

Residents of nursing facilities develop pneumonia approximately ten times more frequently than older adults in the general community population. Pneumonia is the leading cause of morbidity and mortality in nursing home residents.

A study that looked at 102,842 nursing home residents in New York, Mississippi, and Maine for a year reported that 3 percent (3085) of those residents experienced a case of pneumonia during the year. Each case of aspiration costs an average of $30,000 in care. While the cause of the pneumonia was not tracked, if one third of the cases were caused by oropharyngeal bacteria, the cost to care for these 1028 cases of pneumonia would be estimated at $30,840,000. If these numbers are extrapolated to reflect the nation's reported 1.5 million nursing home residents, the cost of poor oral care related aspiration pneumonia would reach $450,000,000. With numerous studies showing oral cleanliness prevents pneumonia in vulnerable populations, it only makes sense for Medicaid to fund oral care efforts.

Diabetes is another medical condition that costs Medicaid an enormous amount of money. Consider the facts:

- The number of residents with diabetes was 362,000 or 24.2 percent of residents. Source: 2004 National Nursing Home Survey (most recent survey).

- People with diagnosed diabetes incur average medical expenditures of about $13,700 per year, of which about $7,900 is attributed to diabetes. Source: American Diabetes Association.

- The total number of people with diabetes is projected to rise from 171 million in 2000 to 366 million in 2030. These findings indicate that the "diabetes epidemic" will continue. Source: Diabetes Care 2004.

- In 2013, Medicaid was the primary payer for over 63 percent of nursing facility residents. Source: Henry J. Kaiser Family Foundation

An analysis of these numbers can conclude that Medicaid is spending approximately $1,801,674,000 in direct medical costs as a result of diabetes and another $ 1,322,748,000 in down line medical costs to care for residents with diabetes. This is a total of $3,124,422,000. If effective oral care procedures were put in place and reduced diabetes costs by a mere 3 percent, Medicaid would save approximately $93,732,660. When the savings of pneumonia care and diabetes care alone are combined, Medicare could potentially save approximately $544,000,000.

Of course, oral care services come with a price. It is nowhere near the cost of caring for folks with aspiration pneumonia and diabetes. Services to keep oropharyngeal bacteria from causing illness can be delivered for $1,200 annually per resident. Oral care services to the 228,060 residents with diabetes who Medicaid funds would cost Medicaid $273,672,000. If Medicaid would fund oral care services for residents who contract aspiration pneumonia, the cost would be $18,000,000. This would still result in a savings of $252,328,000 and oral care services are likely to reduce cost by more than what is projected here.

Insurance Companies

Not all residents' medical costs are covered by Medicaid. There are approximately 37 percent of residents who rely on traditional insurance or their own finances to cover nursing home costs. Insurance companies are beginning to see a value in improved oral health.

- In 2010, Cigna Insurance published report of a $2483 savings in down line medical costs in people with diabetes who had periodontal treatment. Delta Dental offered increased dental hygiene benefits to those with diabetes, renal failure, chemotherapy, and cardiovascular disease.

- In March of 2013, United Healthcare published a paper

showing that their subscribers who had dental hygiene treatments saved thousands of dollars a year especially if they were non-compliant in treating their primary illness, from Asthma to Cardiovascular disease.

With findings such as these, the findings reflected in other published research, and the numbers discussed in the Medicaid section above, it makes complete sense to move toward funding oral care efforts in the elder population insurance companies support.

Nursing Homes

The U.S. Department of Health and Human Services (HHS) 2014 budget proposal included a package of Medicare legislative proposals that could save $371.0 billion over ten years. Changes to the Affordable Care Act will impose penalties towards nursing facilities by refusing to pay for unplanned readmissions to hospitals within thirty days for complications to specific conditions including heart attacks, heart failure, and pneumonia. An analysis by the Medicare Payment Advisory Commission indicates that nearly 14 percent of individuals on Medicare discharged from a hospital to a skilled nursing setting are readmitted to the hospital for conditions that could potentially have been avoided. The HHS 2014 budget proposal recommended reducing payments by up to 3 percent for skilled nursing facilities that are determined to have high rates of preventable hospital readmissions. The proposed penalties would take effect in 2017, with an estimated $2.2 billion in savings over ten years from these penalties alone.

Nursing homes need to look at ways to prevent hospital readmissions in order to prevent fines they cannot afford to pay. Improved oral health can help prevent these conditions and hospital readmissions. The investment of providing professional services is a logical to not only reduce readmissions, but to prevent illness that cause hospital admissions in the first place.

Private Pay

There are residents and/or residents' families who are in a position to be able to pay for extra services. Some of the services that are paid for privately are hair care, nail care, massage, etc. These services can certainly assist with quality of life and people are willing to pay for such services. Educating family members about the potential health problems poor oral health can cause, about the inability of the facilities care team to provide adequate oral care, and the challenges around getting dental/dental hygiene services for their loved ones opens their eyes to these issues. Once they understand all of these things, many families will do what they can to ensure their family member receives oral care services.

Chapter Ten

It Is All About the People

This book has focused on many of the aspects of oral care. However, the most important piece of this whole situation is the people. The dependent elders who are suffering needlessly from the condition of their mouths. These are the people who have directly influenced the writing of this manuscript and to who this work is dedicated.

Ed's inability to move on his own, bathe himself, or dress himself landed him in a nursing home at age eighty. Though he did the best he could to take care of his mouth, his condition affected his hands and he was not able to brush effectively. Ed may have traveled down the same path as Gladys, Ida, and Helen, if it were not for a hygienist providing weekly oral care and xylitol.

Weekly oral care visits were enjoyable for Ed and the hygienist. They visited, flossed and brushed, and managed to give each other a hard time now and again. Before long, Ed's gums were healthy and they remained that way, as did his teeth. His gums did not bleed and the plaque on his teeth was very minimal. During the time Ed was receiving oral care services, he was free of dental disease, did not require any treatment from a dentist, and never needed emergency dental care. Ed did not contract any cases of aspiration pneumonia and his diabetes was managed successfully. As Ed's condition deteriorated and as he neared death, the hygienist was present to provide comfort care for his mouth. And while Ed did move on from this world, he did not die from dirty teeth.

George was stricken by Alzheimer's and was placed in the care of a medical team in a memory unit. His wife understood how important George's oral health had been to him throughout his life. She realized he required more help with his oral care than the care team was able to provide. A hygienist was hired to provide oral care services for George. Over the eighteen months these services have been being provided, George has had no cavities. He has however broken several teeth, which the hygienist has been able to facilitate the repair of at a local dental office. She has gone so far as to accompany George and his wife to the dental visits. She has been able to communicate George's needs to the dental team. Even though his physical and mental conditions continue to deteriorate, he has not had pneumonia or been hospitalized. Even though George is for the most part, nonverbal he managed to say, "Thank you" to the hygienist after she brushed and flossed his teeth during a recent visit. This incident brought tears to the eyes of the nurse who witnessed his words.

Elaine's daughter realized the care team working in the memory unit were not able to provide the level of assistance with oral care she needed, because her mother would not allow them to help. A hygienist was hired to perform the ADL of tooth brushing and between the teeth cleaning. Elaine allowed the hygienist access to her mouth from the first day they met. Elaine had a root that had decayed under a crown. The hygienist noticed it while flossing. Elaine's daughter was notified. Elaine was taken to the dentist and the tooth was removed. This prevented the situation from becoming an emergency.

Charlie was nearing death and his wife noticed his mouth was full of debris and plaque. A hygienist was hired to provide oral care services. While Charlie was uncooperative with his wife and the care team during oral care, he did not resist the hygienist when she brushed and cleaned between his teeth. Over the three months the hygienist cared for Charlie, she also provided support and friendship to his wife. A couple days before Charlie passed away the hygienist saw something happening that she had never seen before. She asked a nurse to look to see if she knew what it was. The nurse put her hands up in the air and said, "I don't do saliva" and would not get close enough to see what was happening. The hygienist went home and began to contact her colleagues to find out what it may have been. The nurse probably never thought about it again.

In conclusion, hygienists need to be providing oral care services to elders who cannot perform adequate oral care measures for themselves. This is necessary to not only prevent dental disease, but to ward off incidences of pneumonia, uncontrolled diabetes, COPD, heart disease, stroke, and dementia. The sequelae of oral disease have been recognized by many influential people and groups, including the U.S. Surgeon General, American Academy of Periodontology, and the American Diabetes Association. Those who are not familiar with the magnitude of what poor oral health can lead to, think oral care should be the task of the nursing assistant, while others feel providing professional oral care would come at too large of cost. These are common misconceptions. Therefore, the hope for this book is twofold. First, it is hoped that it has presented enough evidence for readers to understand the price of proper prevention is much less than paying the price to treat conditions caused by dental disease and the price is not only measured by money. Secondly, and most importantly, it is hoped readers understand elders have, and will continue to, die from dirty teeth until massive action is taken.

Despite many obstacles, I am taking massive action. I am the hygienist who provided oral care services to Ed and Charlie and who is currently caring for George and Elaine. Gladys, who was mentioned in the first chapter, was my mother-in-law and Helen was my grandma. Their suffering from dental disease contributed to their death and I was only able to watch it happen. I have made them a promise that I will not remain silent again. It has taken me many years to understand what is happening and to develop a protocol that can help. If you have a loved one who needs help with oral care, get them help. If you are a medical or dental professional and work with this population, be sure their oral care needs are being met by someone who can manage those special needs. I am preventing our elders from dying from dirty teeth. So can you.

Appendix A

Facts About Xylitol

Information supplied by and reprinted with permission from xylitol.org

When was xylitol discovered?

Xylitol was discovered almost simultaneously by German and French chemists in the late 19th century and has been used extensively in Europe since World War II. Its dental significance was researched in Finland in the early 1970s, when scientists showed it had significant dental benefits. In Finland, Sweden, Japan and many other countries, xylitol is widely used in candy, gum and oral care products. While xylitol is fairly new in the US market, its use is rapidly increasing as more people become aware of its unique health benefits.

What is Xylitol? How can I find products with xylitol?

Just visit our products section. As an educational website, Xylitol.org provides information about a wide range of products that contain xylitol. Our rating system shows which products contain sufficient amounts of xylitol to be effective and all-natural ingredients.

Is it possible to replace daily teeth cleaning with xylitol usage?

A healthy mouth and teeth are an important part of vigorous everyday life. That is why it is important to take good care of them. To keep a beautiful and healthy smile brush your teeth daily and visit your dentists regularly.

How much xylitol should you use?

Xylitol is a natural and convenient way of supplementing daily dental care. Research shows that a mere 6g to 10g day is enough. Xylitol should be chewed immediately after a meal or a snack. If you eat more snacks, you of course need more frequent help from xylitol.

How long does the protection last?

Studies show the xylitol effect on teeth is long-lasting and possibly permanent. Low decay rates persist even years after the trials have been completed. In addition to starving harmful bacteria of their food source, use of xylitol raises the pH of saliva in the mouth. When pH is above seven, calcium and phosphate salts in saliva start to precipitate into those parts of enamel where they are lacking. For this reason, use of xylitol has demonstrated not only a dramatic reduction in new tooth decay, it also has shown the arrest and even some reversal of existing dental caries.

Why does xylitol help protect teeth from cavities?

Sugar feeds bacteria in your mouth, causing them to multiply rapidly. This metabolic process produces acids that cause cavities to begin to form. When you use xylitol gum or mints, the acid attack that would otherwise last for over half an hour is stopped. Because the bacteria in the mouth causing caries are unable to ferment xylitol in their metabolism, their growth is reduced. The number of acid-producing bacteria may fall as much as 90 percent. Since no acid is formed, the pH of saliva does not fall. See more at: http://xylitol.org/about-xylitol/faqs-questions-about-xylitol#sthash.JctYtfu5.dpuf

Can diabetics use xylitol?

The body does not require insulin to metabolize xylitol. For this reason polyols like xylitol produce a lower glycemic response than sucrose or glucose. This has made xylitol a widely used sweetener for the diabetic diet in some countries. If you do have diabetes, however, it's important to consult your doctor or diet professional before incorporating xylitol into your daily diet.

Is xylitol toxic to dogs?

Many dog owners are aware that chocolate, coffee, and grapes are toxic to dogs, but are unaware of the risk from ingesting the common natural sweetener, xylitol. Xylitol is a natural sweetener that is found in a variety of products, including chewing gum, toothpaste, mints, floss, candy, chewable vitamins, and sugar-free baked goods. While xylitol offers many health benefits to humans, it can be deadly to dogs and should not be fed to any pets.

Ingesting 100 milligram of xylitol per kilogram of bodyweight may cause a rapid release of the hormone insulin, causing a sudden decrease in blood glucose (potentially life-threatening hypoglycemia, low blood sugar) for dogs. The drop in blood sugar occurs within fifteen minutes, while the symptoms of hypoglycemia (vomiting, depression, loss of coordination, seizures, or coma are all possible symptoms) may be seen within thirty minutes after the dog consumes the xylitol-containing product. Exposure to higher doses of xylitol may possibly result in fatal liver failure in some dogs.

Is it dangerous to swallow gum with xylitol?

No, it is not — but xylitol chewing gum, like other chewing gum, is not meant to be swallowed. If it does get swallowed, it will be transported naturally among other food through intestines. The best way to dispose of your chewing gum is to wrap in a piece of paper and throw it in a waste basket.

What are the other health benefits of xylitol?

First, you are doing your body a big favor by substituting more xylitol for sugar in your diet. While xylitol is just as sweet as table sugar (sucrose), it has about 40 percent fewer calories and 75 percent fewer carbohydrates. Xylitol also won't raise your blood sugar like regular sugar does, putting tremendous strain on your system, causing negative health effects.

Xylitol has also been proven to inhibit the growth of bacteria. Research shows that this effect enables xylitol to help prevent bacteria and irritants from adhering to upper respiratory passages when used as a nasal wash. Studies have also shown that 8 grams of xylitol, taken orally every day, prevented about 40 percent of ear infections. For more information on these and other benefits, visit our medical section.

Benefits Overview

Xylitol serves as an effective sugar substitute for diabetics and non-diabetics. Xylitol use also provides excellent dental benefits. Using xylitol has many benefits:

- Delicious sweet taste with no unpleasant aftertaste

- Helps reduce the development of dental caries

- Reduces plaque formation

- Increases salivary flow to aid in the repair of damaged tooth enamel

- Provides one third fewer calories than sugar

- May be useful as a sugar alternative for people with diabetes (on the advice of their healthcare providers)

Xylitol Dental Benefits

Studies using xylitol as either a sugar substitute or a small dietary addition have demonstrated a dramatic reduction in new tooth decay, along with arrest and even some reversal of existing dental caries. This xylitol benefit is long-lasting and possibly permanent. Low decay rates persist even years after the trials have been completed.

It's 100 percent natural.

Xylitol is not an artificial substance, but a normal part of everyday metabolism. Xylitol is widely distributed throughout nature in small amounts.

It's safe.

In the amounts needed to prevent tooth decay (less than 15 grams per day), xylitol benefits and is safe for everyone. The World Health Organization has given xylitol its safest rating for food additives.

It's convenient to use.

Xylitol can be conveniently delivered to your teeth via chewing gum, tablets, or even candy. You don't need to change your normal routine to make room for Xylitol.

It tastes great.

One of the best xylitol benefits is its great taste. Xylitol is a health regimen that doesn't require iron willpower or discipline. Xylitol tastes so good, using it becomes automatic, for both adults and children.

How to Use Xylitol

It is not necessary to replace all sweeteners to get the dental benefits of xylitol. Look for xylitol sweetened products that encourage chewing or sucking to keep the xylitol in contact with your teeth. The best items are 100 percent xylitol. Next best are items where xylitol is the principal sweetener. Always make sure there are no acids in the products.

How much Xylitol should I use?

The older research with xylitol always specified an amount 6-10 grams as being the "sweet spot." Newer research has actually shown better how to use xylitol, and that the quantity is not the most important, but the number of exposures throughout the day. We want to get at least four to five exposures of 100 percent xylitol spread throughout the day. When products that contain HSH, sorbitol, maltitol and other sweeteners are used their effectiveness is diminished and you will need to use much more product. Remember that we are trying to "starve" the bacteria, and providing all of those other sugars that feed the bacteria makes the job that much more difficult. So rather than thinking in terms of "how much" think in terms of "how often."

How often should I use Xylitol?

If used only occasionally or even as often as once a day, xylitol may not be effective, regardless of the amount. Use xylitol at least three, and preferably five times every day. Remember the following Strive for Five program:

STRIVE FOR FIVE:

1. Use Xylitol toothpaste, mouthwash, and nasal spray upon waking up

2. After breakfast use Xylitol gum, mints, or candy

3. After lunch use Xylitol gum, mints, or candy

4. After dinner use Xylitol gum, mints, or candy

5. Use Xylitol toothpaste, mouthwash, and nasal spray upon going to bed

When should I use Xylitol?

Use immediately upon waking up in the form of toothpaste and mouthwash. If you drink tea or coffee in the morning use xylitol to sweeten it. After breakfast use a candy or chewing gum with xylitol. After lunch use a few pieces of gum or candy, and then again after dinner. Before going to bed in the evening be sure to brush with xylitol toothpaste and use a xylitol mouthwash. There is a dental floss available with xylitol that helps get it in between the teeth.

Remember that throughout the day any time you would normally use chewing gum or eat candy make sure you are using xylitol sweetened products. There is an increased benefit up to six to seven times a day.

RESOURCES

Photos from the case studies can be found at: http://hylifellc.com/studyphotos

Research and statistics found in this book are from the following sources:

American Dental Hygienists' Association. "Direct Access." http://www.adha.org/direct-access.

American Diabetes Association. "The Cost of Diabetes." (Last Updated: April 18, 2014). http://www.diabetes.org/advocacy/news-events/cost-of-diabetes.html.

Assisted Living Federation of America. "Nursing Homes May Face Readmission Penalties Similar to Hospitals." (Last Updated: April 16, 2013). http://www.alfa.org/News/3102/Nursing-Homes-May-Face-Readmission-Penalties-Similar-to-Hospitals.

Carter, Pamela. *Lippincott's Textbook for Nursing Assistants.* (Philadelphia: Wolters Kluwer Health/Lippincott Williams & Wilkins, 2012).

Centers for Disease Control and Prevention. *FastStats: Diabetes.* (Last Updated: January 7, 2015). http://www.cdc.gov/nchs/fastats/diabetes.htm.

Centers for Disease Control and Prevention. *National Diabetes Statistics Report: Estimates of Diabetes and Its Burden in the United States, 2014.* (Atlanta, GA: U.S. Department of Health and Human Services, 2014). http://www.cdc.gov/diabetes/pubs/statsreport14/national-diabetes-report-web.pdf.

Cigna. "Improved Health and Lower Medical Costs: Why good dental care is important." 2010. http://ktbenefits.com/uploads/Medical%20and%20Dental%20with%20Cigna.pdf.

Delta Dental. "Delta Dental PPO Plus Direct Plan." http://www.ehealthinsurance.com/ehealthinsurance/benefits/dt/DT-CO-DeltaPPOPlusDirect-1009.pdf.

Furman, Christian Davis, Abi V. Rayner,and Elisabeth Pelcher Tobin. "Pneumonia in Older Residents of Long-Term Care Facilities." *American Family Physician* 70, no 8(2004 Oct 15):1495-1500. http://www.aafp.org/afp/2004/1015/p1495.html.

Goldberg, Larry. "Medicare and the FY 2014 budget." (McGladrey: 2013). http://mcgladrey.com/content/dam/mcgladrey/pdf_download/medicare_fy2014_budget.pdf.

Henry J. Kaiser Family Foundation. "Overview of Nursing Facility Capacity, Financing, and Ownership in the United States in 2011." (June 28, 2013). http://kff.org/medicaid/fact-sheet/overview-of-nursing-facility-capacity-financing-and-ownership-in-the-united-states-in-2011.

Langmore, Susan, Kimberly Skarupski, Pil Park, and Brant Fries. "Predictors of aspiration pneumonia in nursing home residents." Dysphagia 17, no. 4 (2002 Fall):298-307.

Pipes, Sally. "Health Costs Resume Their Rise." Forbes. (May 5, 2014). http://www.forbes.com/sites/sallypipes/2014/05/05/health-costs-resume-their-rise.

UnitedHealthcare. "What's Driving Up Premiums and 6 Ways You Can Lessen the Blow." Health Care Outlook. (October 2013). http://www.uhctogether.com/Mid-a/35900.html.

U.S. Department of Health and Human Services. "Oral Health in America: A Report of the Surgeon General." (Rockville, MD: U.S. Department of Health and Human Services, National Institute of Dental and Craniofacial Research, National Institutes of Health, 2000). http://www.nidcr.nih.gov/DataStatistics/SurgeonGeneral/Documents/hck1ocv.@www.surgeon.fullrpt.pdf.

U.S. Dept. of Health and Human Services, National Center for Health Statistics. "National Nursing Home Survey, 2004." (Hyattsville, MD: U.S. Dept. of Health and Human Services, National Center for Health Statistics [producer], 2004. Ann Arbor, MI: Inter-university Consortium for Political and Social Research [distributor], 2007-03-23). http://doi.org/10.3886/ICPSR04651.v1.

Wolgin, Francie. *Being a Nursing Assistant.* (Saddle River, N.J. : Prentice Hall Health, 2005).

About the Author

Angie Stone has been a dental professional for over thirty years. Her career began serving our great country as a dental technician in the United States Navy. Once she completed her enlistment, she obtained her associates degree in dental hygiene from Madison Area Technical College, Madison, WI and later earned her bachelor of science in psychology from Upper Iowa University. Angie has been the editor in chief of *Hygiene Tribune*, had numerous articles published in a variety of publications, and has authored a chapter in the book *Dare To Be a Difference Maker*. Her original research concerning elders and xylitol has been published in a peer reviewed medical journal. Angie was awarded the Sunstar/RDH Magazine Award of Distinction in 2012 for her work with the geriatric population and xylitol. Angie has presented to dental professionals in thirty-five states and four countries and territories, including Greece, Mexico, Canada and Puerto Rico. She is also a seven time attendee of CareerFusion.

Made in the USA
Middletown, DE
09 July 2022

68697240R00064